I0415536

Lesson One:

STOP

PUTTING

CIGARETTES

IN

YOUR

MOUTH,

LIGHTING

THE

TIPS

OF

THEM

ON

FIRE,

AND

INHALING

WHAT

COMES

OUT

OF

THE

BUTT

END.

FOLLOW

THIS

SIMPLE

STEP

AND

YOU

WILL

NEVER,

EVER

SMOKE

AGAIN,

GUARANTEED!

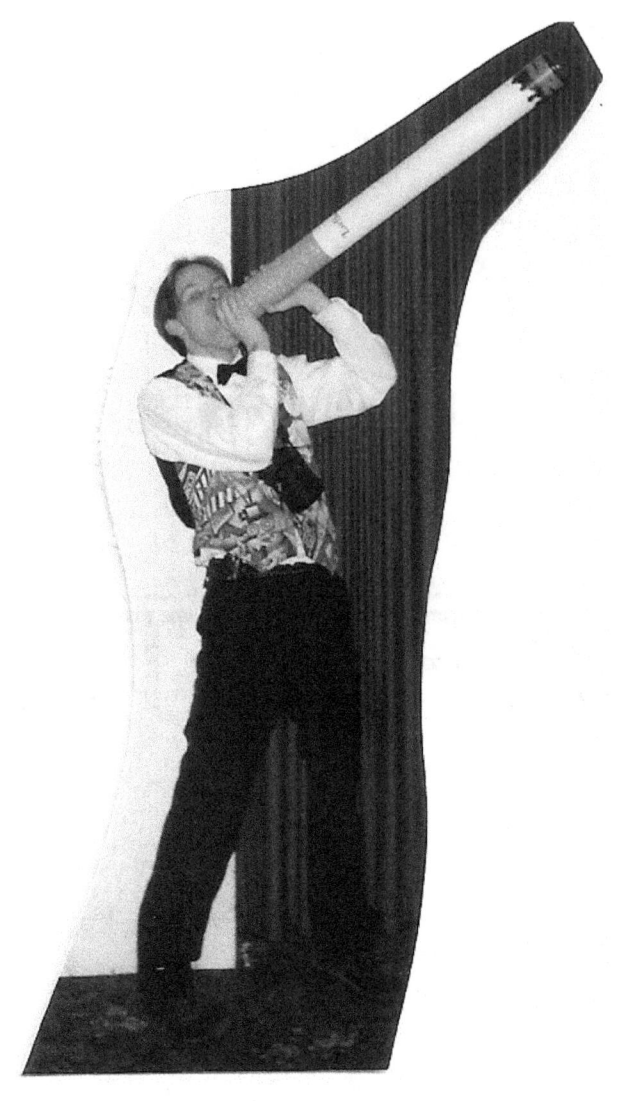

The author, Derrick G. Wood, at work in 1999

www.ingramcontent.com/pod-product-compliance
Lightning Source LLC
Chambersburg PA
CBHW070813290526
45795CB00002B/711